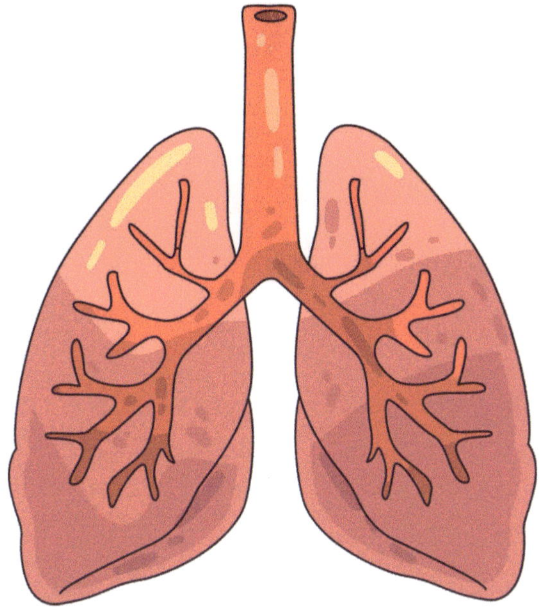

BREATHE HOPE

A COMPREHENSIVE GUIDE TO LUNG CANCER AWARENESS, PREVENTION, AND HEALING

AF679475

Breathe Hope : A Comprehensive Guide to Lung Cancer Awareness, Prevention, and Healing

Copyright © 2025 by Delatria Sam
All rights reserved.
No part of this publication may be reproduced, distributed, or transmitted in any form or by any means, including photocopying, recording, or other electronic or mechanical methods, without the prior written permission from the publisher or author, except as permitted by U.S. copyright law,
ISBN: 979-8-3496-5561-6

With Heartfelt Support

May today's awareness, education, and informative resources inspire proactive steps toward a healthier tomorrow.

This dedication is to:
- Healthcare workers who care tirelessly for those affected by lung cancer,
- Patients affected who face lung cancer with strength and resilience,
-Families, friends, and communities impacted by lung cancer,
- Caregivers who provide love, support, and compassion on this journey,
- And everyone who strives for awareness, prevention, and a healthier future.

What is LUNG CANCER?

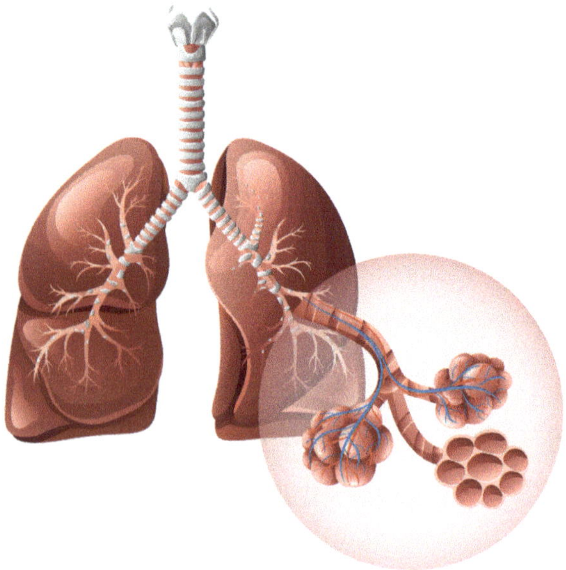

Lung Cancer is a type of cancer that originates in the lungs and can spread to other parts of the body.

Listen to Your Lung's Signals:

- Wheezing
- Shortness of breath
- Recurring Respiratory Infections
- Fatigue
- Chest pain
- Weight Loss
- Loss of Appetite

FINDING STRENGTH: PHYSICAL ACTIVITIES FOR LUNG CANCER HEALING

WALKING: GENTLE WALKS FOR EXERCISE AND FRESH AIR

YOGA: MODIFIED POSES FOR FLEXIBILITY AND STRESS RELIEF

STRETCHING: GENTLE STRETCHES TO MAINTAIN MOBILITY

TAI CHI: LOW-IMPACT MOVEMENTS FOR BALANCE AND GAIT

LIGHT AEROBICS: ADAPTED FOR ENERGY LEVELS

BREATHING EXERCISES: HELP MANAGE SYMPTOMS

CHAIR EXERCISES: SEATED MOVEMENTS FOR LIMITED MOBILITY

SHORT BIKE RIDES: IF ENERGY ALLOWS

LIGHT GARDENING: THERAPEUTIC AND ENGAGING

DANCING: LOW IMPACT, FUN, AND MOVEMENT

PILATES: CORE STRENGTH AND FLEXIBILITY

SWIMMING OR WATER THERAPY: LOW-IMPACT FOR JOINTS

DID YOU KNOW?

Lung Cancer is one of the leading causes of cancer deaths worldwide.

LUNG CANCER WELLNESS HABITS

Stick to your doctor's treatment plan and attend all follow-up appointments.

Learn ways to manage symptoms like breathing difficulties or pain with your healthcare team.

Gentle exercise like walking can help improve mood and energy if your doctor says it's okay.

Focus on a balanced diet to help your body cope with treatment.

Join groups for emotional support and connection with others going through similar experiences.

Try techniques like meditation or deep breathing to help manage stress.

Learn about lung cancer, treatment options, and ask your healthcare team questions.

Get enough rest to help your body recover from treatment and manage fatigue.

Lung Cancer

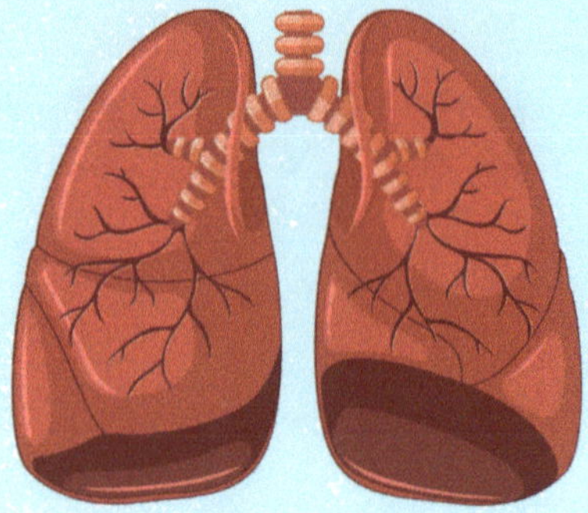

Risk Factors and Prevention

What Puts Pressure on Your lungs?

Smoking and tobacco use, environmental pollutants, and occupational hazards.

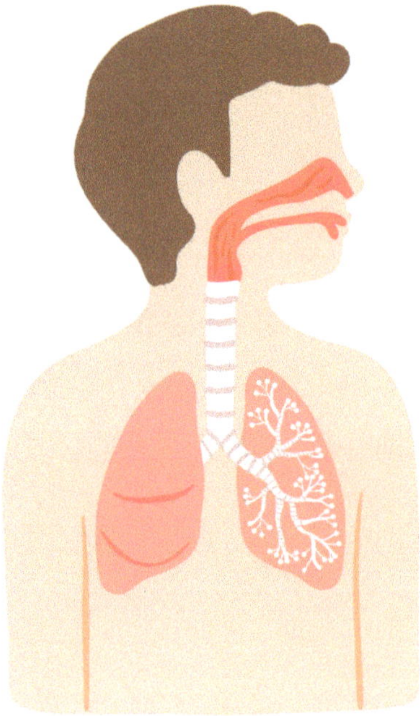

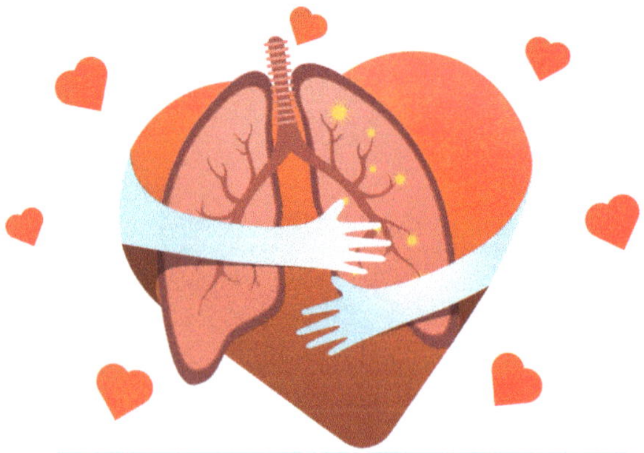

What else can I do to protect my lungs:

Wear protective gear, exercise regularly, stay hydrated, have regular check-ups, and improve indoor air quality.

How Can I Protect My lungs?

- Lifestyle Changes
- Avoiding Harmful Exposures
- Don' t Smoke
- Test For Radon
- Staying Active
- Eating A Healthy Diet
- Staying Informed

TESTIMONIAL

TESTIMONIAL

TESTIMONIAL

"After quitting smoking, I noticed a significant improvement in my breathing and overall health."

Rachel, former smoker

TESTIMONIAL

TESTIMONIAL
TESTIMONIAL

"Early detection saved my life. I encourage everyone to get screened if they're at risk."

John, lung cancer survivor

TESTIMONIAL

"My family's support means everything. We face lung cancer together, one day at a time."

Sarah, patient

TESTIMONIAL

TESTIMONIAL
TESTIMONIAL

"Clinical trials gave me hope when traditional treatments weren't working. It's worth exploring all options."

Michael, lung cancer patient

TESTIMONIAL

TESTIMONIAL
TESTIMONIAL

"I wish I had known about radon testing sooner. Protect your home and your health."

Emily, lung cancer survivor

TESTIMONIAL

TESTIMONIAL

TESTIMONIAL

"

Exercise and a healthy diet have been crucial in my recovery. Small changes make a big difference."

David, survivor

TESTIMONIAL

“Don’t ignore the symptoms. Persistent coughs or shortness of breath should be checked out."

Mark, patient

TESTIMONIAL

TESTIMONIAL
TESTIMONIAL

"Awareness and education are key. Let's work together to fight lung cancer."

Karen, advocate

TESTIMONIAL

"Targeted therapy has been a game-changer for me. Stay informed about the latest treatments."

Lisa, patient

TESTIMONIAL
TESTIMONIAL
TESTIMONIAL

"I'm grateful for every day I have. Lung cancer may be tough, but it's not impossible to overcome."

James, survivor

DID YOU KNOW?

Radon exposure is the #1 cause of lung cancer in non-smokers. Testing your home for radon is a simple step you can take to protect your lung health.

MANAGING LUNG HEALTH

THE DOCTOR'S ADVICE:	THE PATIENT'S CONCERNS & QUESTIONS:
"Hi there! I'm Dr. Barry. I understand you've been having some concerns about your lung health?"	"Yes! I've been a smoker for years and was worried that if I continued long-term, it would be detrimental to my lungs."
"Let's talk about lung cancer risks. Smoking's a major risk factor. If you smoke, quitting's the best thing for reducing risk."	"My uncle was a smoker and got lung cancer. Am I at higher risk due to family history?"
"Family history can slightly increase risk, but smoking's a bigger factor. Given your uncle's history and your smoking habits, we'll monitor your lung health closely."	"That sounds good. What are the benefits of quitting in terms of reducing lung cancer risk?"
"Quitting smoking can reduce your risk of developing lung cancer. The sooner you quit, the better. We'll also discuss screening options to catch any potential issues early."	"Okay, that makes sense. What symptoms should I watch out for? Also, what kind of screening would you recommend?"
"Watch for coughing blood, chest pain, or breathlessness. For screening, we may consider low-dose CT scans. Let's follow up in a few months to reassess and discuss screening options."	"Sounds good, Dr. Barry. I'll make sure to quit smoking and schedule that follow-up."

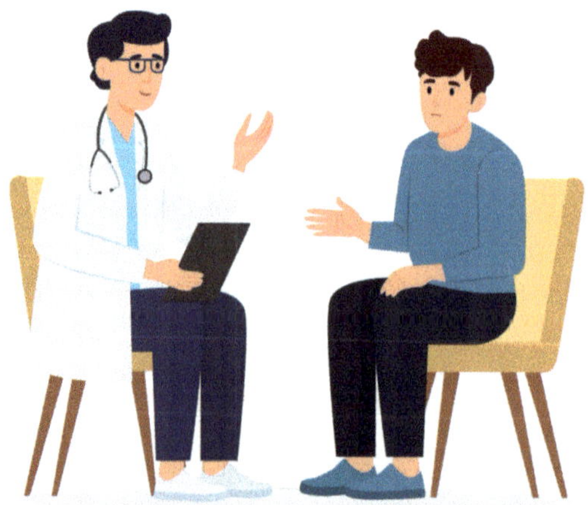

LUNG CANCER AWARENESS:

KNOW THE SIGNS. SAVE LIVES.

Some additional symptoms that you should know about:

LUNG CANCER:

- **Voice Alert:** Hoarseness or changes in your voice
- **Swelling Warning:** Swelling in the face, arms, or neck
- **Swallowing Struggle:** Trouble Swallowing or pain when swallowing
- **Coughing Up:** Coughing up phlegm with rust-colored sputum
- **Persistent Cough Alert:** A cough that doesn't go away or gets worse.

Spreading awareness about these symptoms can help catch lung cancer early. Share this info with your loved ones, and let's fight for lung health together!

BREATHE HOPE

COMMUNITY EVENT

Create a community-driven event to raise awareness about lung cancer, promote prevention strategies, and support healing for those affected.

Activities can include: Lung Health Fair (info booths, healthcare Q&A), Breathe Hope Art (create art/messages for survivors), Survivor Stories (share resilience stories.

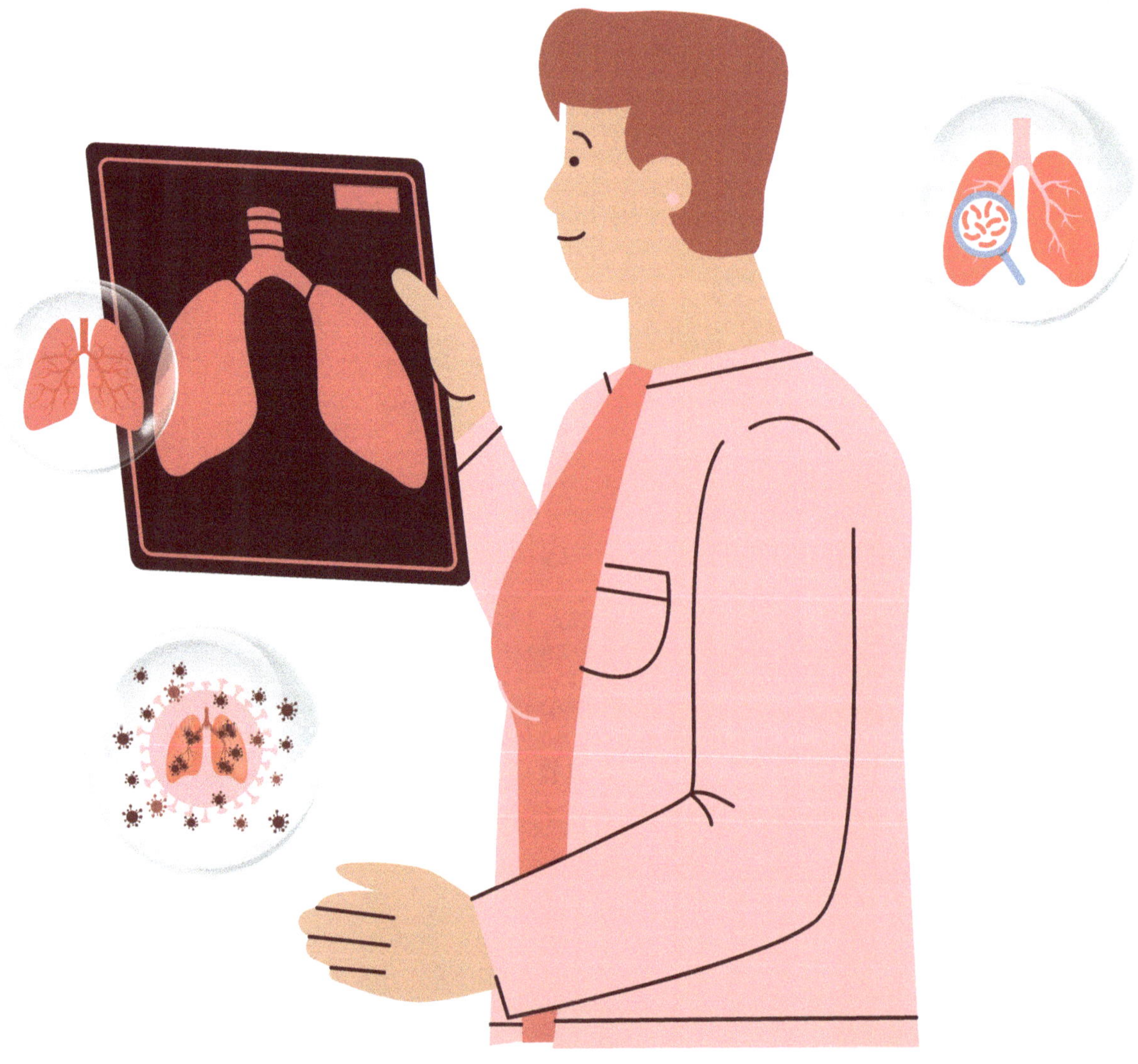

LUNG HEALTH TIPS FOR A HAPPIER YOU!

Love Your Lungs: 6 Tips To Follow

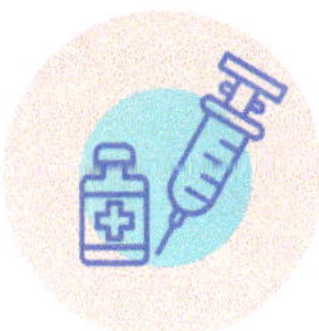

Stay-Up-To-Date on Vaccines: Protect against infections like flu/pneumonia

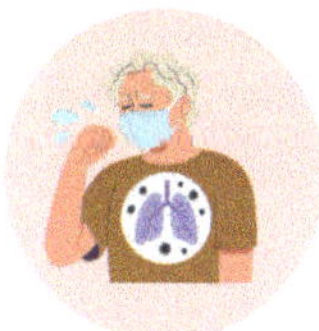

Protect Lungs at Work

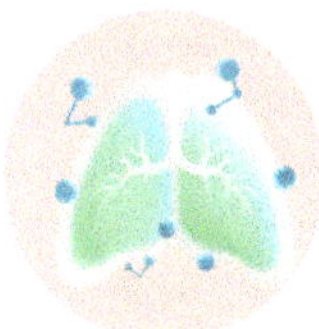

Support Lung Cancer Research

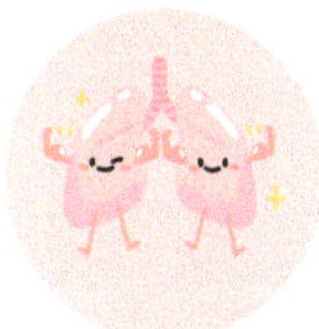

Healthy Lungs=Healthy Body

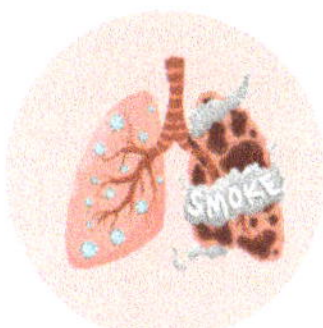

Know Your Risk Factors

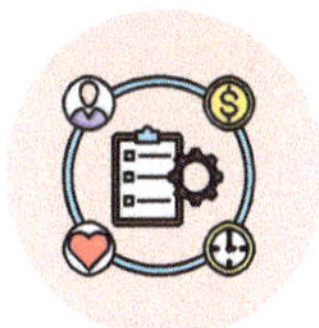

Use Resources like Counseling or Medications to Quit Smoking

BREATHE HEALTHY: THESE PARTS WORK TOGETHER FOR BREATHING AND GAS EXCHANGE.

Study this worksheet. Later, you'll label these parts on the "Lungs Health Challenge" worksheet.

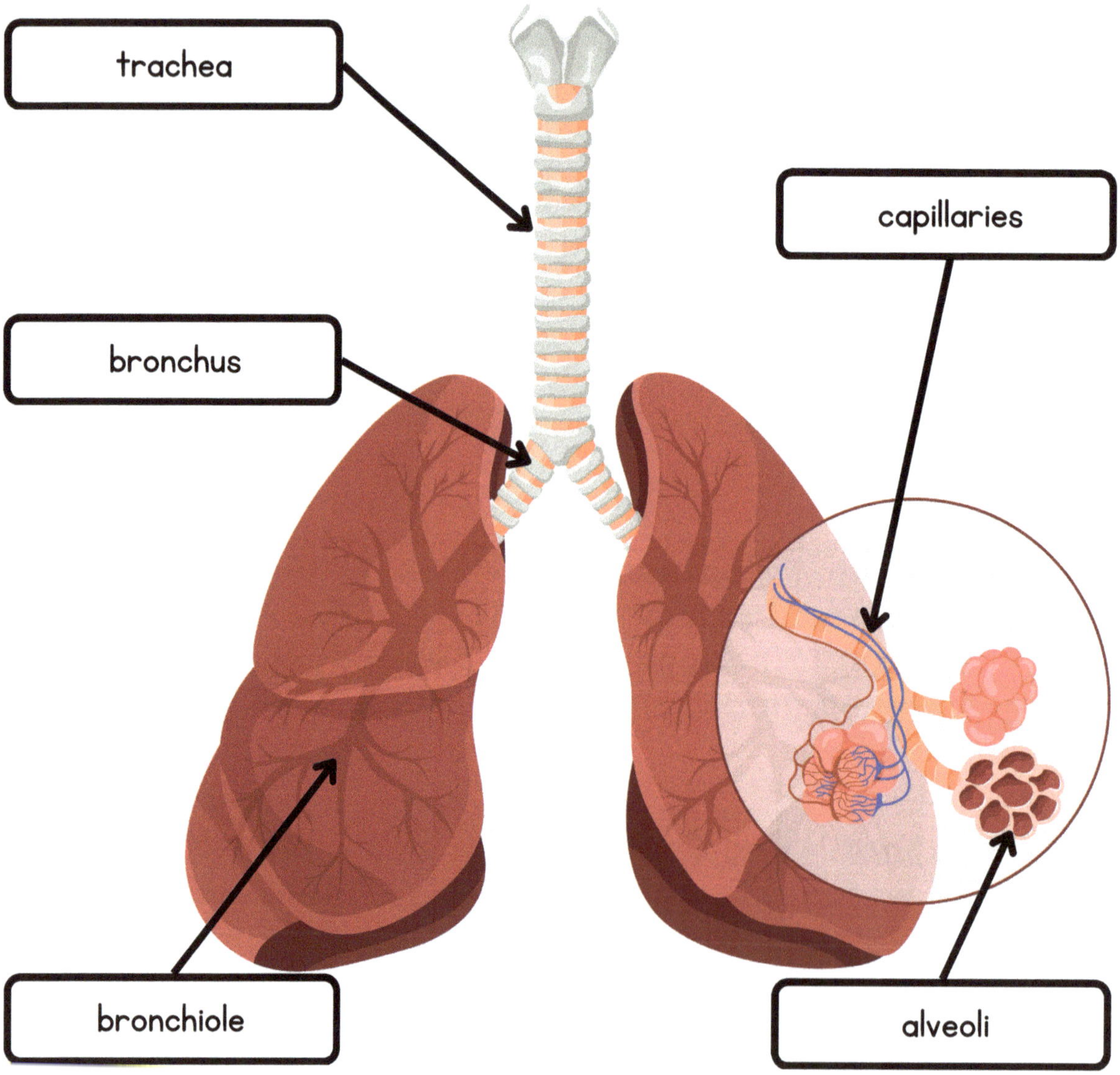

HOPE

STRENGTH

SUPPORT

COURAGE

RESILIENCE

LET'S BE AWARE

We can fight lung cancer together

LEARN THE SYMPTOMS OF LUNG CANCER. **GET CHECKED OUT TODAY** IF YOU'RE AT RISK OR HAVE CONCERNS! VISIT LUNGCANCER.ORG AND SAVEDBYTHESCAN.ORG FOR MORE INFORMATION.

HOW CAN YOU HELP?

- SPREAD AWARENESS ABOUT LUNG CNCER RISKS AND PREVENTION.
- SUPPORT LUNG CANCER RESEARCH AND PATIENTS.
- SHARE THIS ACTIVITY WITH FRIENDS AND FAMILY.

Words of Courage

May these words be supportive for those affected by lung cancer.

1. Stay Strong!
2. Be Brave!
3. Find Hope!
4. Keep Fighting!

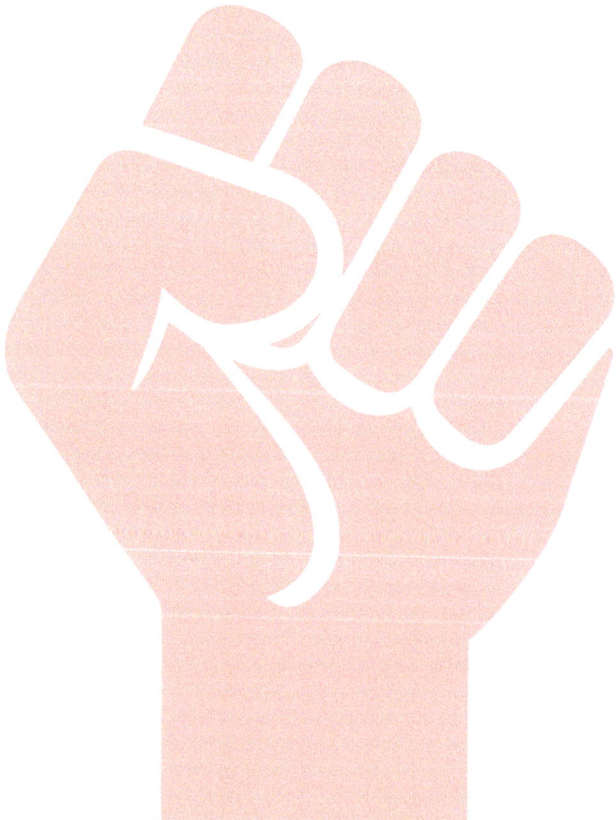

Sharing Your Story

This space is for you to share your story, thoughts, and feelings about lung cancer. Whether it's your own journey or someone close to you, we encourage you to reflect on your experiences and share what you've learned along the way.

My lung cancer journey

A good day with lung cancer

Challenges I've faced

Sources of strength

Lessons Learned

Hope for the future....

What I'd like others to know about lung cancer

LUNG HEALTH CHALLENGE

Label the Lungs. After labeling, write a personal pledge on the sticky note on the next page about one thing you can do to promote lung health.

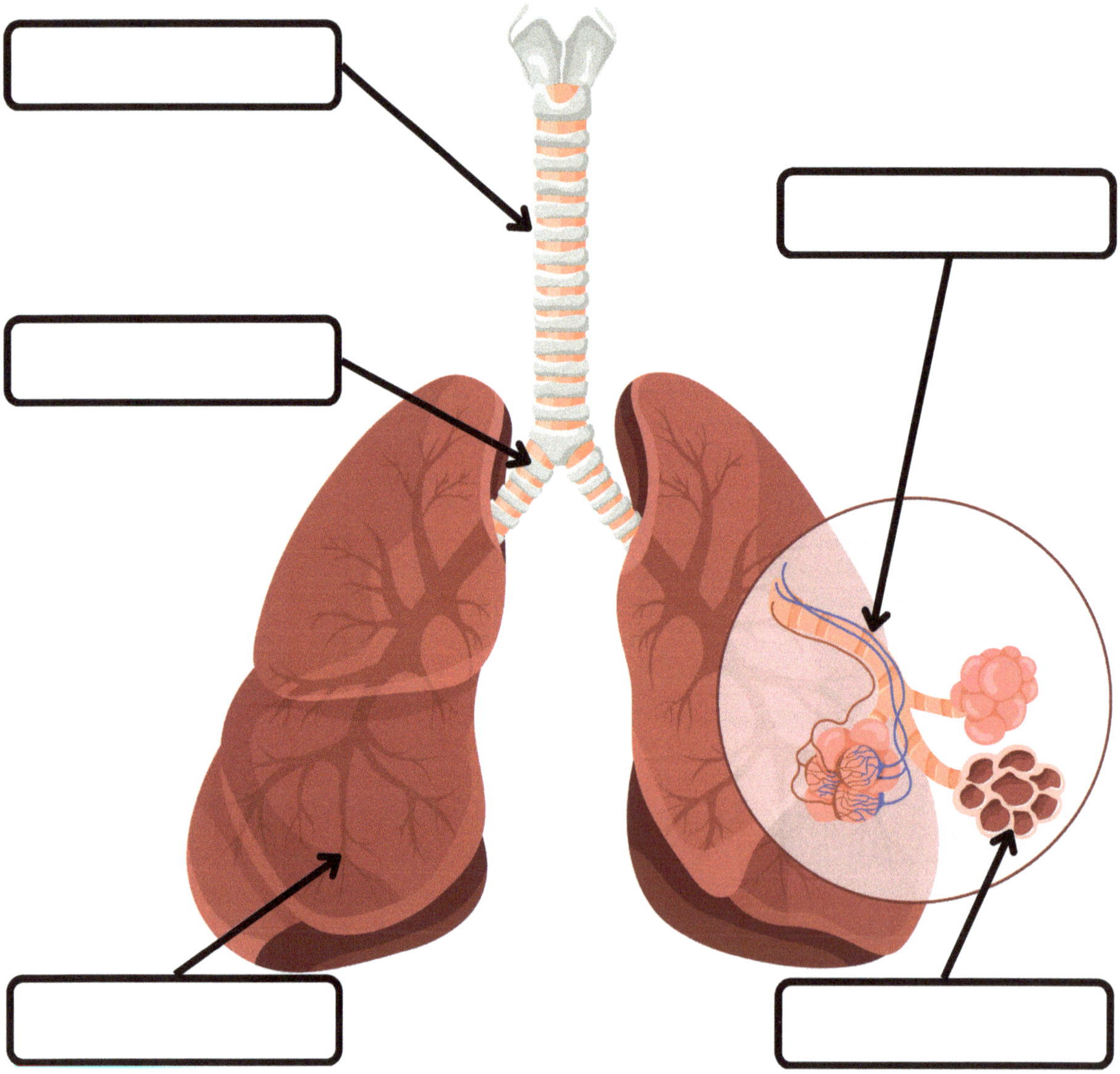

capillaries   trachea   bronchus   bronchiole   alveoli

MINI-QUIZ

NAME ONE RISK FACTOR FOR LUNG CANCER?

MINI-QUIZ

HOW DOES QUITTING SMOKING IMPACT LUNG HEALTH?

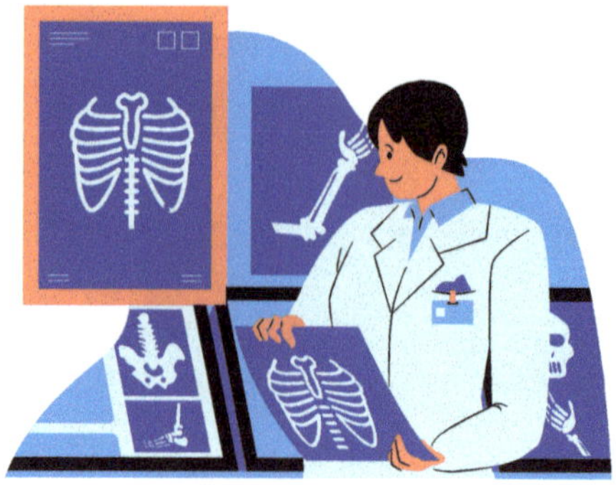

How might Lung Cancer be diagnosed?

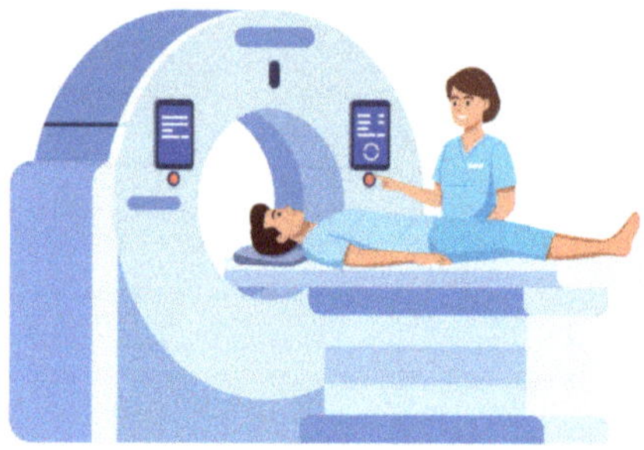

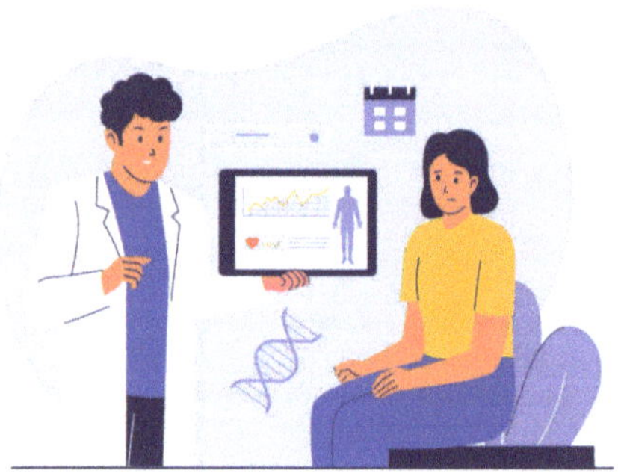

Diagnosed:

- **Medical History and Physical Exam:** A doctor evaluates symptoms, risk factors, and overall health.
- **Imaging Tests:**
  - Chest X-ray: Identifies abnormalities in the lungs.
  - CT Scan: Provides detailed images of the lungs and surrounding tissues.
  - PET Scan: Helps determine if cancer has spread.
- **Biopsy:** A tissue sample is taken from the lung tumor or affected area for examination.
- **Sputum Cytology:** Mucus is examined for the presence of cancer cells.
- **Bronchoscopy:** A flexible tube with a camera is inserted through the mouth or nose to visualize the lungs and collect tissue samples.

DID YOU KNOW?

Radon exposure is the second leading cause of lung cancer.

Love Letters

My Partner Fighting Lung Cancer

"My love, every breath you take is a testament to your strength. I'm here for you, always, and I'll fight alongside you."

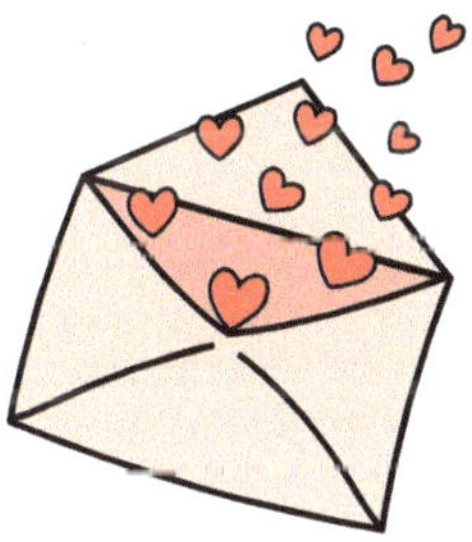

To My Loved One Who Lost Their Battle

"My dear, I'll never forget the memories we shared. Your love and legacy live on in my heart."

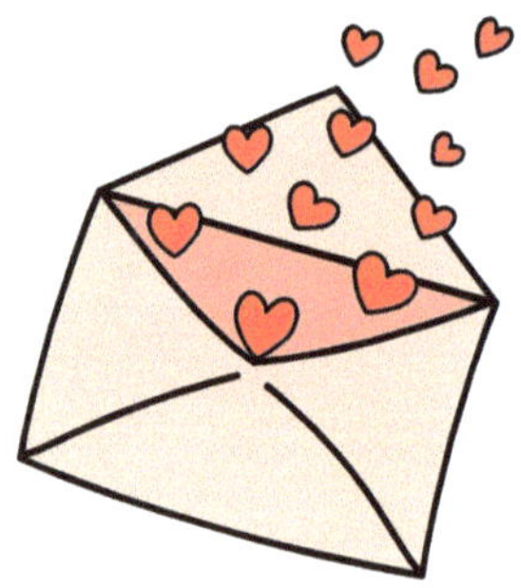

To a Friend Newly Diagnosed

"Dear friend, I know the words 'lung cancer' can be overwhelming. But I want you to know you're not alone. I'm here for you."

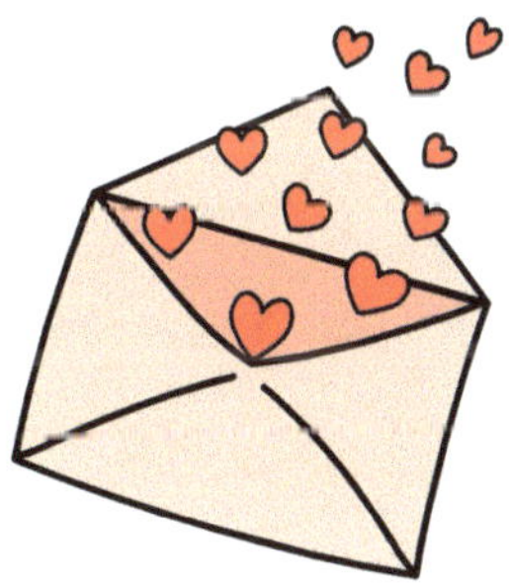

To My Caregiver

"Dear caregiver, your love and support mean everything to those fighting lung cancer. Thank you for being a source of strength."

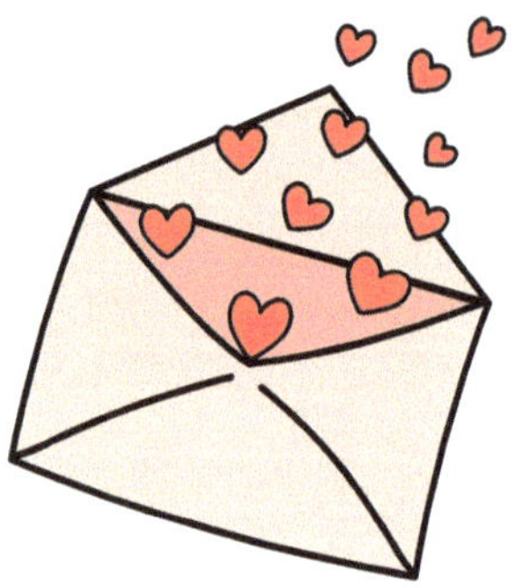

To Myself During Treatment

"Dear self, this journey may be tough, but you're tougher. Keep pushing forward, even on the hardest days."

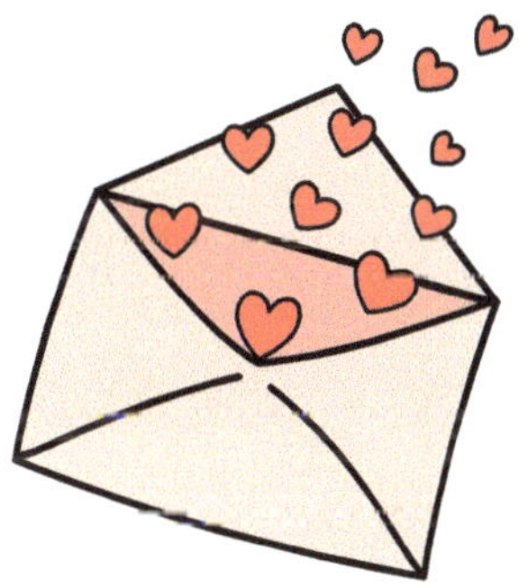

To Those Who Have Lost Loved Ones to Lung Cancer

"I'm so sorry. May the memories of your loved ones bring you comfort and peace."

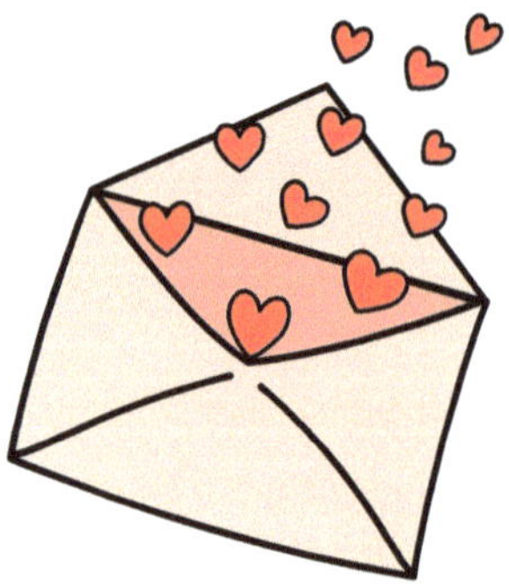

To A Survivor

"Your strength inspires me. Your love for life is contagious, and I'm grateful to know you."

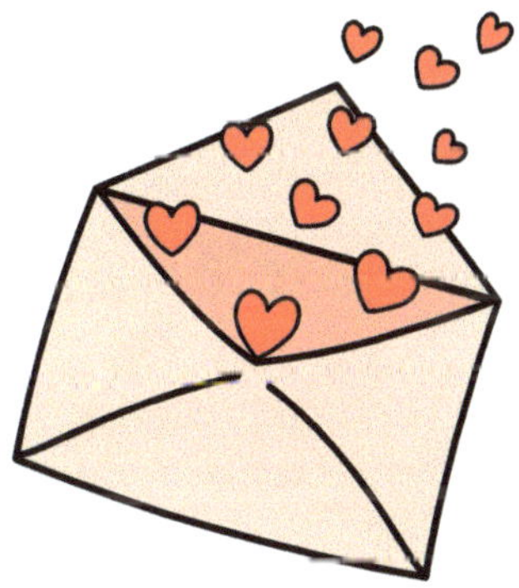

To Those Who Are Still Fighting

"Dear friend, you're not alone in this fight. Keep pushing forward, even when it feels like the darkness is overwhelming."

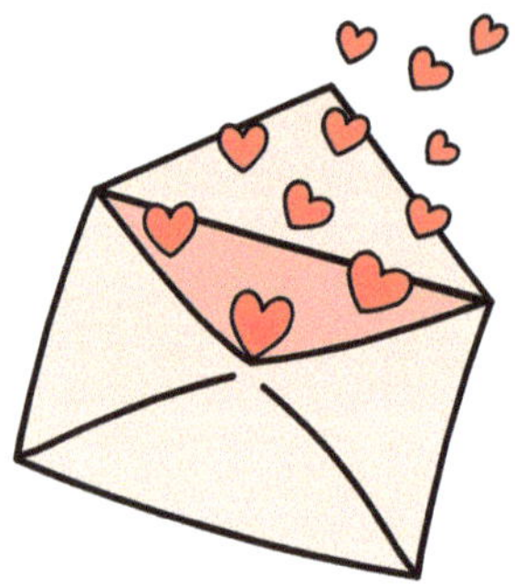

To the Doctors and Nurses

"Dear medical team, thank you for your tireless efforts to care for those affected by lung cancer. Your compassion and expertise are beacons of hope."

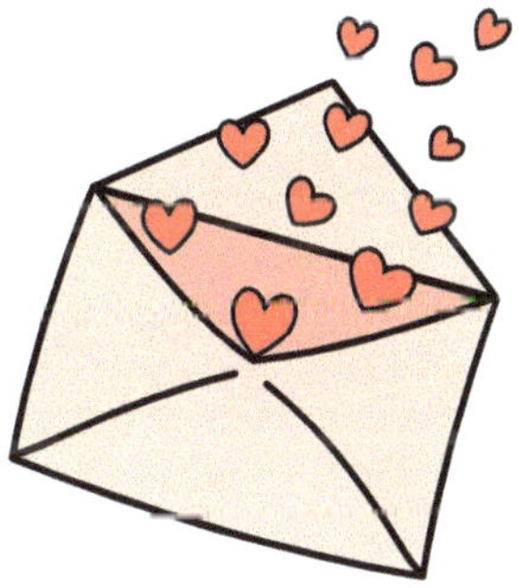

To Hope

"You are the light that guides us through the darkest times. Thank you for being a constant companion on this journey."

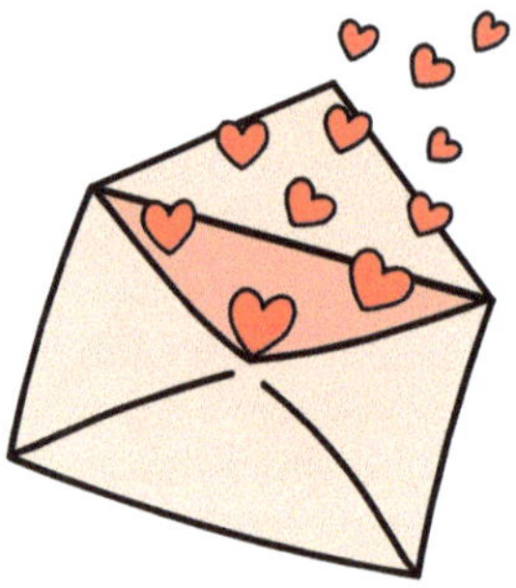

DID YOU KNOW?

Some people who have never smoked can still develop lung cancer, and in fact, lung cancer in non-smokers is on the rise.

Q&A Time

QUESTION

What are the most common causes of lung cancer?

ANSWER

The most common causes are smoking, followed by exposure to carcinogens like radon, asbestos, and air pollution.

What are some other ways to help spread awareness?

- ☐ Share lung health tips on social media
- ☐ Organize a community walk or run for lung health
- ☐ Host a healthy-lung class
- ☐ Volunteer at a local health fair
- ☐ Talk to friends and family about lung cancer risk factors
- ☐ Share personal stories or experiences with lung health
- ☐ Participate in lung cancer awareness campaigns
- ☐ Encourage others to get regular check-ups
- ☐ Distribute lung health brochures or flyers
- ☐ Support organizations focused on lung cancer research and awareness

DID YOU KNOW?

Advances in targeted therapy and immunotherapy are improving treatment options for lung cancer patients, offering new hope for better outcomes and increased survival rates.

Q&A Time

QUESTION

Who should get screened for lung cancer?

ANSWER

Current or former smokers aged 50-80, or those with a family history.

DID YOU KNOW?

Lung cancer can affect anyone, regardless of age, smoking history, or background.

Q&A Time

QUESTION

What are the potential side effects of lung cancer treatment?

ANSWER

Common side effects include fatigue, nausea, hair loss, and shortness of breath, which can vary depending on the treatment type.

THOUGHTFUL IDEAS FOR SOMEONE AFFECTED BY LUNG CANCER

gift list

Cozy blanket	Relaxation Music
Soft pillows	Portable Oxygen tank Holder
Comforting tea or coffee gift basket	Humidifier
Aromatherapy essentials	Emergency contact list
Personalized journal	Gift Card for Grocery Delivery
Photo album	tablet or E-Reader
Comfortable socks	Inspirational quotes wall art
Warm hat or scarf	Air purifier
Stress ball or fidget toy	Personalized care package
Inspirational book	Comfortable clothing
Cozy Slippers	Personal care items
Support group information	Pill organizer
Portable water bottle	Customized sympathy card
Healthy snack basket	Nutritious Food Basket

DID YOU KNOW?

Some studies suggest that a diet rich in fruits, vegetables, and whole grains may help reduce the risk of lung cancer, even for smokers.

Q&A Time

QUESTION

How can I support a loved one with lung cancer?

ANSWER

Offer emotional support, help with daily tasks, and encourage them to seek professional help when needed.

How To Talk To Someone With Lung Cancer

PERSON A

"Hey, how are you doing? I've been thinking about your lung cancer diagnosis. How's everything going?"

PERSON B

"It's going okay, thanks for asking. I'm managing my symptoms and trying to stay as comfortable as possible."

PERSON A

"That's good to hear. What does your doctor say about managing symptoms? Are there things you're supposed to avoid?"

PERSON B

"Yeah, I'm supposed to avoid things that could irritate my lungs more. I'm trying to stick to what my doctor recommends."

PERSON A

"Makes sense. Do you need help with anything, or want to talk about how you're handling everything?"

PERSON B

"Thanks for offering. Just checking in is nice. It helps knowing people care."

DID YOU KNOW?

Protecting yourself and others from secondhand smoke can be a lifesaver.

Q&A Time

QUESTION

What are the benefits of participating in lung cancer clinical trials?

ANSWER

Clinical trials provide access to new treatments, contribute to medical research, and may offer additional treatment options.

LET'S DO A LUNG CANCER MYTH-BUSTERS CHALLENGE!

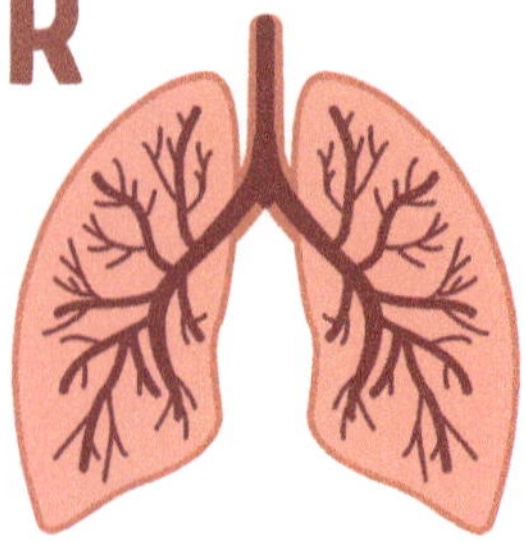

Test your knowledge about lung cancer. Fill out the below.
Bonus: Create an awareness tweet using the facts you learn #LungCancerAwareness

WHAT I KNOW	WHAT I WANT TO KNOW	WHAT I LEARNED

LUNGS EXPLORER ACTIVITY: BREATHE EASY!

Learn about lung structure, function, and how to keep lungs healthy.

What do the lungs look like? Draw or describe the lungs and their parts (bronchi, alveoli, etc).

What are the functions of the lungs? Explain how lungs help with oxygen, carbon dioxide, and overall health.

What is the lung made up of? Explore and list the various parts of the lungs and their respective functions.

LUNGS ADVENTURE: LABEL & DISCOVER!

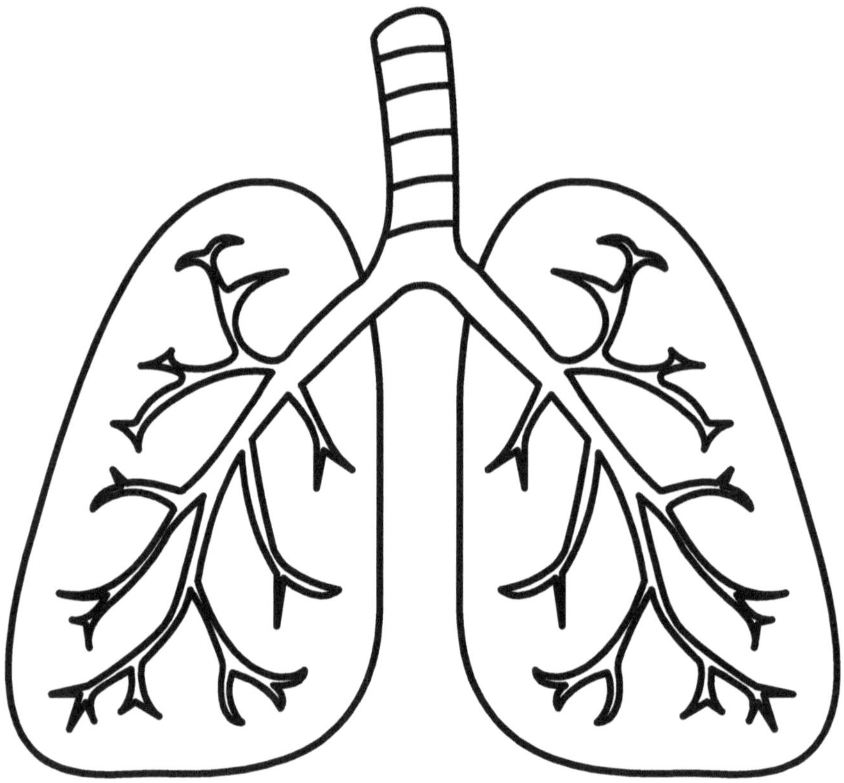

Label the lungs diagram: Trachea, Bronchi, Bronchioles, Alveoli.
Describe each part's function.
Bonus: How can you keep your lungs healthy?
Wrap-Up: Share what you learned about lungs!

Q&A Time

QUESTION

Where can I find resources and support for lung cancer?

ANSWER

Organizations like the American Cancer Society, Lung Cancer Foundation, and online support groups offer resources, information, and at local community events.

Q&A Time

QUESTION

How can I talk to my family about lung cancer risk?

ANSWER

Be open and honest about your concerns, share information about risk factors, and encourage them to talk about their concerns with a healthcare provider.

LUNG HERO!

WHAT DO YOU REMEMBER ABOUT HOW TO LOWER YOUR RISK OF LUNG CANCER? WRITE DOWN ACTIONS IN EACH BUBBLE THAT PROMOTE LUNG HEALTH AND REDUCE LUNG CANCER RISKS.

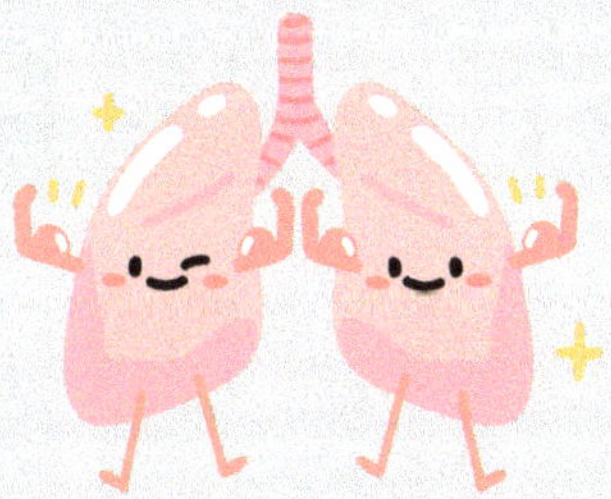

Research Update

Clinical Trials are exploring new therapies, such as tarlatamab and zongertinib, for small-cell lung cancer and NSCLC.

Source: ClinicalTrials.gov

Q&A Time

QUESTION

Can lung cancer recur after treatment?

ANSWER

Yes, lung cancer can recur, which is why follow-up care and monitoring are crucial.

Discover the Power of Early Detection!

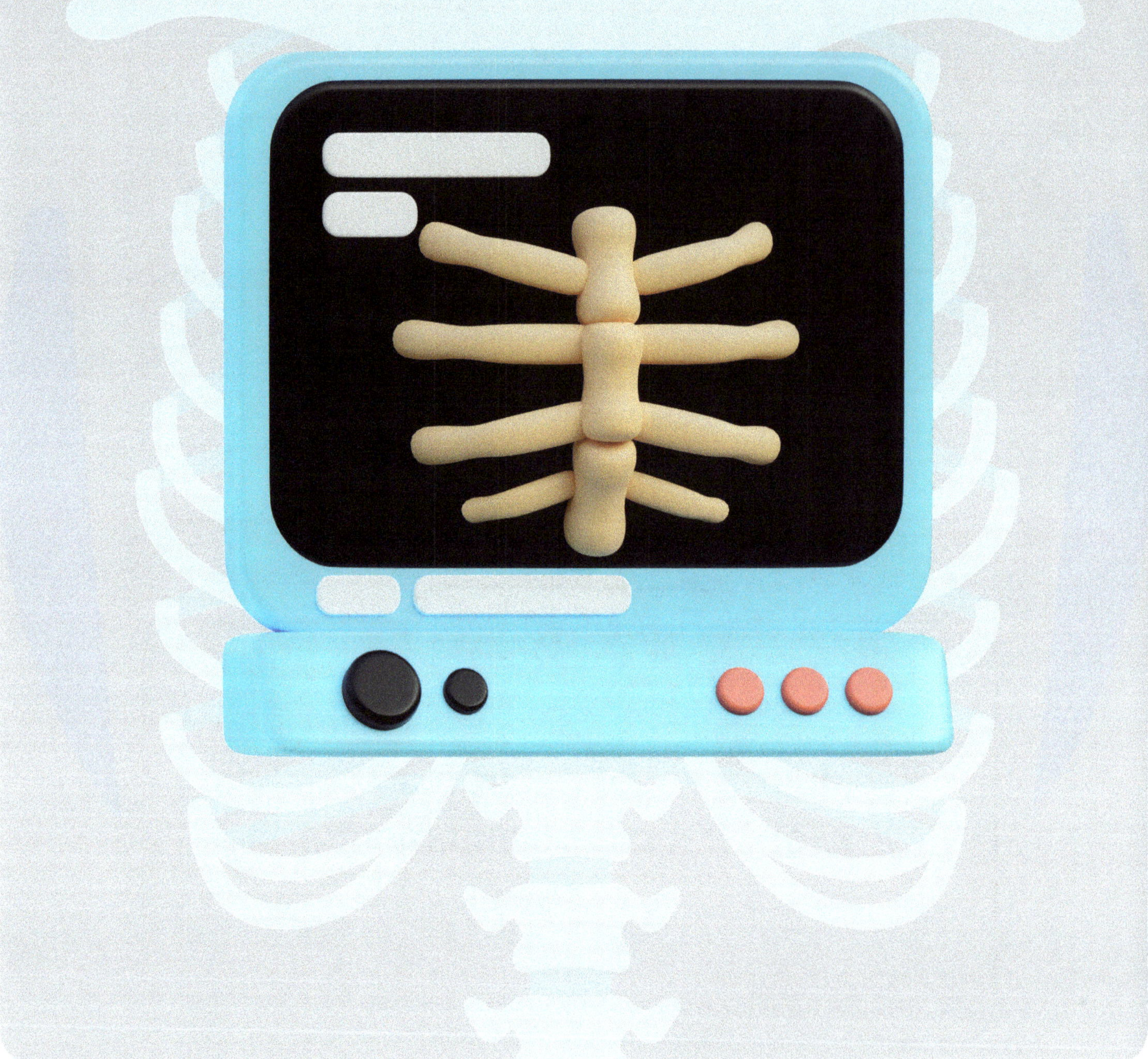

Chest X-rays help spot lung issues before symptoms show up.

- Take Charge of Your Lung Health! A simple chest X-ray can reveal a lot about your lungs.
- See Clearly, Breathe Easily! Early detection of lung issues means better outcomes.
- Know More About Your Lungs! Chest X-ray screenings are a step toward proactive health care.

Q&A Time

QUESTION

What are some key questions to ask my doctor about lung cancer treatment?

ANSWER

Questions might include: What stage is my cancer? What treatment options are available? What are the potential side effects? What are the chances of success?

Medical Glossary

These terms can help understand key concepts and terminology.

Adenocarcinoma	A type of non-small cell lung cancer.
Lung Nodule	A small growth on the lung.
Pleural Effusion	Fluid buildup in the space around the lungs
Lobectomy	Surgical removal of a lung lobe.
Pneumonectomy	Surgical removal of an entire lung.
Non-Small Cell Lung Cancer (NSCLC)	The most common type of lung cancer.
Small Cell Lung Cancer (SCLC)	An aggressive type of lung cancer.
Lung Cancer Staging	Determining the extent or spread of lung cancer.
Metastasis	Cancer spread from the lungs to other parts of the body.
Thoracotomy	Surgical incision into the chest cavity.
Pulmonary Function Test	A test to measure lung function.
Radiation Pneumonitis	Inflammation of the lungs due to radiation therapy.
Targeted Therapy	Treatment targeting specific lung cancer cell characteristics.
Biomarker	A substance used to detect or monitor lung cancer.
Lung Cancer Screening	Tests to detect lung cancer in high-risk individuals.